I0441769

KEEPING HEALTH SIMPLE

Sleep, exercise, diet, positive thoughts, and nervous system supply. These are the five areas of health that will be discussed in this book. You are most likely familiar with the first four concepts, but the importance of maintaining your nervous system may be a new idea for you. As a doctor of chiropractic, I have realized the importance of "the master system" that controls the body. More on that later!

The real purpose of this book is to demystify health information. There is so much out there with the new age of data. Articles fly across the internet at light speed, and often times one article will conflict with the other. Consumers are confused, and rightly so! Hopefully the information contained within these pages will help you look at each bit of information through a specific lens-the lens of physiological design!

What is physiological design? I believe that the human body was made to perform a particular way. Whether you believe in evolution or not makes no difference. Either through intentional creation or natural selection our bodies were made to function a certain way. We are made to eat certain foods, drink certain liquids, sleep, think, and move certain ways. The Western world is facing a crisis in healthcare, and it all stems from the fact that our daily habits have taken us too far from our intended design. This book will remind you to think about physiologic design when making choices about your health.

Does this seem too easy? After reviewing countless studies related to a wide variety of diseases, I have come to the conclusion that optimal health is really not difficult to achieve.

The first step in reclaiming your health is to realize you are your own best doctor. You know more about your body than any person on the outside ever will. Consider two important ideas: 1. Your health is your responsibility. 2. You understand your body better than anyone else on the planet. Once you accept responsibility for your health and realize that you are your own best doctor, the journey can begin!

Before I get into specifics, I would like to tell you a little bit about how I arrived in the field of health care. Hopefully this background information will help you understand why I have come to these conclusions about health and how you can use the tips in this book to start your journey towards optimal living.

Like most people, it took a negative event to begin my search for optimal health. When I was in my mid-twenties I was still teaching elementary school when I developed a pain in my left side. At first I thought it was just indigestion from the cafeteria food, but the pain not only persisted, it got worse. I went to my medical doctor, who was more holistic than the typical M.D. She asked me about my diet and when I described my typical meal, her eyes got as big as half-dollars! Back then I was a huge meat-eater who had two grills and used them almost every weekend. Generally half of my plate was either chicken, beef, or pork. She quickly diagnosed me with diverticulitis and advised me to cut down the amount of meat on my plate to less than 25%. I did and I immediately felt better! The pain went away after just a few days and I was amazed that I "cured" myself simply by changing my diet.

That started the health food craze that I have been on for over a decade, and I feel amazing! That pain in my side led to a cascade of events that has changed me forever. I didn't stop at decreasing my meat intake to less than 25%; I continued to change my eating habits. The next step was to eat a salad for lunch every day. I quickly noticed that my body began to crave salads for lunch, even on the weekends. That was a key point in time for me, because I realized that the body becomes accustomed to whatever you are feeding it, so to make a change you simply have to "push through" a couple of weeks until your body adapts to the change.

Shortly after my salad addiction I decided to start growing my own vegetables. To this day I enjoy maintaining a garden and I can attest that there is no better feeling than eating a meal that you grew yourself. I became fascinated with the world of gardening. Composting, vermicomposting (keeping worms), soil mixtures, and the list goes on and on. I started a garden at the school as well as a recycling program. I was completely engrossed with trying to live healthy while making as little impact on the environment as possible.

Some days instead of eating with the other teachers in the lounge I would stay in my classroom and watch Ted Talk videos. On those days I just needed a few moments alone, and if you have ever been in a classroom with 25 little humans, you know what I'm talking about! On one faithful day I stumbled across a video by Graham Hill entitled: Why I'm a Weekday Vegetarian. In the video he explained how abstaining from meat five days out of the week had the potential to make global changes if enough people started doing it. It was perfect timing! I was already a self-proclaimed salad addict, I was getting into gardening, and I was trying to set the example for the kids I was teaching so that they could live rich and healthy lives as well.

I instantly noticed positive changes in my body. I started waking up easier, with more energy. I didn't "crash" after lunch the way I used to, and by the time I got home from school I still had the drive to go outside and play with my kids! Life was great, but I was still suffering from allergies seasonally. In fact, over the next few years and into my early thirties, my allergies began to spiral out of control.

I began to suffer from sinusitis. Starting around age 30 I would come down with a sinus infection in the fall and one in the spring. Within three years that number had more than doubled. I was coming down with a sinus infection 4-6 times a year, and most of the time had to rely on antibiotics to resolve the infection. Again I went to the medical doctor for answers. She gave me the usually nasal sprays and decongestants but nothing seemed to prevent the infections. So I was referred to an allergist.

I went through the test where they stick you with 50 needles, each one dipped in a different substance to look for an allergic response. I only tested positive for one common allergen...dust mites. I immediately thought of my classroom at school, where a thin film of dust could develop in a matter of days. When you put 25 little humans in a room together, sloughing off skin all the day, dust formation is inevitable. The allergist said there were basically two options: prevention and allergy shots. I knew that prevention was basically impossible given my work environment; I was bound to encounter dust there. So I inquired as to the allergy shots. He informed me that it was a series of weekly shots that spanned over a year. Hmmm...I thought. That sounds like a lot of time and money. I asked what the success rate was. He told me it was about 50%. I raised an eyebrow, very skeptical at this point. Then he informed me that there was a risk associated with the shots, and that in fact 1/1000 people who undergo the treatment die. Come again?!? Did you say 1/1000 people DIE doc? He seemed surprised that I was so shocked. I politely declined the treatment and ran like hell.

Perhaps I overreacted, and I'm no statistician, but a 1/1000 chance of death with only a 50% success rate for the treatment sounds like a bum deal. I consider this event the next turning point in my personal journey towards health, because it was the experience that turned me towards "alternative medicine".

I began to research on my own outside of the conventional medical model. At the same time I went a little bit crazy at home. I ripped all of the carpet out of my house, took down the curtains, and bought all new hypoallergenic everything. Bed sheets, pillows, mattress, etc. Nothing helped. So I switched tactics. Instead of going outside in, I began to focus on inside out. This is a very important concept and as I later discovered a central tenet of chiropractic philosophy. I didn't know it at the time, but I was already beginning to think like a chiropractor.

I began to exercise. And I don't mean twice a week, I am talking about a daily routine. I started a program at school three days a week where I opened up the gym an hour before classes started and led an exercise program for kids with ADHD. (As an aside, the results were amazing and I am currently conducting a research project associated with that program) After school I would go to the gym and lift, even on the days that I exercised in the morning. Some weeks I would get in 7-10 workouts before the weekend started. My professional life was great; as you can imagine the parents of the children were extremely grateful for my initiative. I was looking great too, but my allergies didn't get better, in fact they got worse.

That summer I developed yet another sinus infection. I went to my M.D. and she prescribed antibiotics. I was working out seven days a week and started the P90X program, which was intense to say the least. I was drinking a gallon of water each day, eating fresh vegetables directly from my garden, and getting plenty of sleep. Yet the infection persisted...June, July, and into August. I went back to the doctor and she diagnosed me with chronic sinusitis. I was given a stronger antibiotic and sent home. I finished the antibiotics and I was still sick, you can imagine how upset I was. I started researching chronic sinusitis and discovered it is classified as a low-grade autoimmune disease. My body was attacking itself from the inside out. I felt like I was doing everything right but I just couldn't kick this infection. I didn't know where to turn next.

I had a good friend who had recently graduated from Parker University and was starting his practice as a doctor of chiropractic, so I decided to make him part of my healthcare team. This was the next turning point in my life, and in my opinion the most critical point of the journey. He explained the way the nervous system functioned and how it had the potential to affect every organ, tissue, and cell in the body. I had never heard anything like that before. He recommended that I go see a chiropractor close to me (he was in another city at the time), and to go often. The first few weeks he said I should go 2-3 times a week, and once I have a break through to start cutting back my visits until I was getting checked by the chiropractor once a week.

I took his advice, and it changed my life. All of the other pieces were in place, but apparently I had a compromised nervous system. A misalignment in my spinal column, which the chiropractor calls a subluxation, was interfering with my body's ability to function properly. You can probably guess the rest of the story. After just one week of adjustments, my infection broke. The school year started and I finished my last year teaching. I spent that year enjoying the last portion of my first career and preparing for my next adventure-chiropractic school. The amazing transformation that I experienced was something I had to investigate further.

My hope is that this introduction has shed some light as to how I have arrived at where I am today. Now I will go through some of the specific details that I have come to recognize as key pieces in my own journey. We will be using the perspective of intended design to keep it simple, logical, and natural. If you can use any of this information to improve the quality of your life then my mission is accomplished!

Chapter 1: SLEEP

Could you use a little more sleep? In today's "go-go-go" society, I think everyone could benefit from a few extra hours of rest. Why is sleep so important? It is a time for your body to repair itself, to take a break from the strains of the upright position, and to integrate all of the experiences that you have had that day.

Enter the lens of physiological design...try to imagine the sleeping habits of our early ancestors. Surely they had fire and could keep the night alive as they pleased, but does it make sense for them to do that? Early survival for our species was like a careful chess game, where every move could mean life or death. Think about it: why would you expend extra energy gathering more wood just so you could stay up late and party?

I propose to you that our ancestors went to bed shortly after the sun went down and arose with the sunrise. It only seems natural that they would have adopted this strategy for survival. Our natural circadian rhythms support this theory! It just makes sense from a survival standpoint.

As mentioned in the introduction, before studying to become a doctor, I was an elementary educator. I spent nine years teaching third and fourth grade to a great group of students. During my tenure I was able to witness first hand the difference in cognition between students who had good sleep patterns and those who did not. You would be surprised at the correlation between learning disabilities and sleep patterns. I could write a book on that point alone.

I was blessed my first two years of teaching to have a brother and sister in my classes who were an absolute joy to teach, Monica and Isaac. The first year Monica was in my class and the next year Isaac followed in her footsteps. As you can imagine I got to know the family very well over those two years, between all of the conferences, awards ceremonies, and informal conversations before and after school. Near the end of the second year I commented to the father about what an honor it had been to teach both of his children. I told him how they both always came into class smiling and happy each day. He then told me the secret ingredient to his parenting success-sleep! He put his kiddos to bed at 6:00 every night, and they slept until 6:00 in the morning faithfully! With twelve hours of rest every night, it is no wonder these two outperformed their peers!

A few years later I had moved from general education to special education. This particular school year I had a young man named Johnny who captured a special place in my heart. Johnny was different; there was no doubt about that. He had several diagnoses and a lot of problems to work through. Often he came in with his hair in a mess, looking tired and grumpy. On those days he would usually have a breakdown mid-morning, crying and screaming. The vice principal would have to come and pull him out of the classroom.

Academically, math was especially difficult for him, but he was an excellent reader. Throughout the school year I found ways to relate to him that reading and math were similar in that there was a formula to each subject, and once you mastered the formula it was easy! I really think he just needed someone to believe in him, as is the case with most troubled children. Johnny began to gain confidence as we worked together and by the end of the year he not only passed the state standardized test, he aced it!

Before his success on the test that year, I began to understand the root cause of his problems, which in turn helped me to understand how to help. I arrived early each day to check my emails and set up my classroom, and this day I had received an email from Johnny's mother. It read, "Dear Mr. Murray, I regret to inform you that Johnny chose to stay up until 2:30 a.m. last night playing video games, so he will probably be very tired today." My first thought was: why didn't you go into his room and take the gaming console?!? Instead of arguing with Johnny's mother I simply replied that I understood, thanked her for letting me know, and told her that I would allow Johnny to rest his head if he needed to. I am not sure what portion of Johnny's academic problems could be attributed to his lack of sleep, but I know it was a major factor. The point is, get your kids to sleep as early as possible, and get to bed yourself!

Now I understand that families cannot be in bed by 6:00 p.m. every night. After school activities and work schedules can get in the way. Some nights you will get yourself and your kids to bed later than you might like. That being said, I would encourage you to try to get at least 8-12 hours of sleep every night, and if you are not coming close to those numbers, look at ways to do things differently. I have no doubt in my mind that our bodies were designed for at least 8 hours of sleep each night!

The following information is for the person that just can't seem to find a way to fit in more than 6 hours of sleep Monday-Friday. I understand how hard it can be as a single parent (or even someone in a two-person household) to get the minimum of 8 recommended hours. Scientists say that you can't catch up on sleep, but I am a scientist and I disagree! In the graduate program at Parker University I took on average 24-26 credit hours each semester. Some days I was on campus 16 hours studying with my classmates, and we had to be back at school at 7:00 a.m. again to take the test! As you can imagine some nights I didn't get much sleep. Whenever possible I kept Saturday mornings open so that I could sleep in. I would wake up feeling refreshed and reenergized. Although it goes against the scientific data, I recommend catching up on sleep whenever possible. If you don't get enough during the week try to make time for sleeping in, and naps on the weekend. Physiologically we were designed to get sleep-and plenty of it. Do your best to fit in as many hours as possible.

Chapter 2: EXERCISE

There is one misconception about exercise that most people believe, and that is that you lose weight by exercising. For the most part this is not true. If you believe that you can lose weight by exercising more, it is my opinion that you have been given poor information. Changing your eating habits is the only way to lose weight. Can you burn off some extra calories and fat by exercising? Yes, however, you can never exercise your way out of a poor diet.

Consider the following example. You eat a snickers bar with your lunch. Do you know how long you need to work out to compensate for those extra calories and sugar? Two hours riding a bike. Let's be honest for a moment. Who has two hours to work out every day? I know I don't and I doubt many of you do either.

Hopefully you see the error of believing that you can exercise your way into a new dress or pant size. When I was in undergraduate study at Texas State University, I would go to the gym several times a week to workout. Every time I went to work out I would see my friend Lauren. I am not exaggerating when I tell you that she was there every time I went to workout. When I arrived at the gym she was already red-faced from running on the treadmill or lifting weights. I would do my routine, which usually lasted about an hour, and then I would leave. Lauren was still there every time as I left. I would joke with her and ask, "Do you live here or something?" She told me that she tried to workout 2-3 hours every day. Now I know what you are thinking, she must have looked like a super-model with all of that exercise…right? Actually, Lauren was a bigger girl. She carried it well and was very good looking, but she never could get the weight off. The situation baffled me for years until I came to understand that no matter how many hours a day you exercise, there is no way to compensate for a poor diet. Case and point, I often saw Lauren at the fraternity houses or local bars drinking beer and eating the standard food for college kids: pizza, hamburgers, and French fries. Even with her exercise program that bordered on insanity she couldn't outrun her diet.

At this point you are probably thinking that I am anti-exercise, but this couldn't be further from the truth! I just think it is extremely important that you understand the real value of exercise. You have to know why you are doing something and understand the true benefits to appreciate its value. If you exercise to lose weight and don't see rapid results (which you won't) then you may become frustrated and quit. It is my intention to show you the true value of exercise and encourage you to do it for the right reasons.

As I mentioned before, as a chiropractor I believe that the nervous system is the most important system in the body. With that in mind, I have come to realize that the real benefits of exercise are related to nervous system stimulation. Increased immune function, increased energy, and decreased stress are the true benefits of exercise and a result of nervous system stimulation, in my opinion.

I'm sure each and every one of you reading this book has either gone through a period in your life where you exercised religiously or at least you know someone who has. Did you notice a difference in the way you felt during this time in your life? You probably slept better, felt like you had more energy, and fell sick less often than you normally did in the past. These are the real reasons you should value exercise and include it into your daily routine.

Consider the intent of our design, how often do you think we should exercise? Simple answer there…every day and tons of it. Hunting and gathering food, hauling fuel to keep the fire going, building and repairing shelter, and the list goes on and on. Our bodies were designed to walk long distances every day, run in short bursts (to catch our prey and avoid predators), bend, twist, carry moderate weight, etc. Our bodies were designed to move in such a way.

I am sure you have heard this common phrase before- motion is life. We were made to move around! With our increasingly sedentary lifestyle, it is no wonder that we are sicker than ever as a society. We were not made to sit all day. Unfortunately in school we are "trained" to sit down for hours upon hours and keep quiet and still. This is unnatural and not good for our health.

Now that you know my opinion on exercise, let me give you some specifics about what to do and how to do it. I will give you some steps to follow that I consider easy to accomplish for anyone and a few helpful tricks that could change your life.

First and foremost, walk, walk, walk. As I mentioned before, I believe we were designed to walk throughout the day. I try to walk at least a mile every day, and sometimes I get up to 5 miles. This is a simple exercise that anyone can do, and the best part is-it's free! You can do it anytime in any place, regardless of where you are. Start with a few minutes a couple of times a week and work your way up as you feel comfortable doing so. Your ultimate goal should be to walk at least one mile every day. Make it a family exercise! On the weekends and evenings, instead of driving to the park I walk with my kids. The half-mile journey to the park is extra exercise for me and the kids don't mind at all! Often times we find sticks, interesting rocks, and other cool things on our way. It is a great way to learn about nature, bond as a family, and get some vitamin D!

As far as exercised is concerned, this is likely the most valuable tip I can give you: if you can afford a treadmill, buy one. If your family will allow you to put it in the living room, do it. Some interior decorators may scoff at this idea, but you could always wheel it into the garage before your next dinner party if you are worried about how it will look. The reason I want you to place the treadmill in the living room is to eliminate any excuse for using it. With it right there in the family room, you can use it while the kids are playing, watching television, etc. There is no reason why you couldn't walk during one television show, and eventually try to work up to walking for an hour each day! You will find out very quickly your body will adapt and start to crave your daily walk. You will become addicted to the new level of health!

As a student in a very demanding doctorate program, I learned very quickly that exercise was one way I could keep my body healthy and my mind sharp. Sitting in the classroom from 7 a.m. until 5 p.m. was not very conducive to great health. One of my goals during my time at Parker University was to come out healthier than I entered. Similar to the phrase, "Never trust a skinny chef!" I believe you should not put your faith in an unhealthy doctor. I made a commitment to my own health during my time at the University, and the treadmill was a big part of that pact.

There were many times that I felt I just couldn't sacrifice a whole hour to exercise when I could be studying, but I felt like I would go absolutely insane if I didn't get up and move around a little. So I came up with the idea of studying while I was working out. The only way that I found to be effective was to walk on the treadmill and read or look at flashcards. An amazing thing happened-my grades went up! I noticed that the material I studied while walking on the treadmill seemed to stick in my mind better; I was able to recall much more of the information from my exercise study sessions. And it wasn't just me observing this phenomenon!

17

Friends of mine would see me studying on the treadmill and would often join me. We would get out our notes and walk and ask each other questions. After the test, every single time someone studied with me in this manner they would tell me how much they remembered from our exercising study sessions! Just like sleep, exercise improves mental function and stimulates the nervous system.

Many of us have jobs that require us to take work home with us. Teachers bring home stacks of papers to grade, lawyers read over cases, and people involved in business are constantly reviewing material for meetings and presentations outside of the office. Why not combine exercise with work that needs to be done outside of the home? I think you will find that the information you review on the treadmill will stick with you longer.

An important part of developing healthy habits is to impress upon your children how important it is. Combining exercise and study is a great strategy to pass on to your kids. Why not quiz your kids with flashcards as you walk to the park? Their test scores will go up and they will be developing healthy habits that last a lifetime.

You can also combine your personal development goals with your workouts. Often times I enjoy walking around the neighborhood practicing one of my presentations as I stroll. I simply print out the power point slides before I go and walk and talk to myself. My neighbors might think I'm a little off the wall but I'm ok with that! If I do not have a public speaking event in the near future I use that time to listen to something informational or motivational. Exercising feels great, exercising and growing as a person feels amazing! I have also noticed that time seems to slip away as you walk with the intention of practicing a speech or listening to a motivational speaker. I tend to keep walking until the speaker is finished or until I feel that I have mastered my talk. Often times this amounts to 3 miles or more and over an hour of exercise.

Just a few words about high-impact exercises and excessive weight lifting. First of all, it isn't natural to do it often. I'm sure that our early ancestors carried loads of moderate weight on a regular basis; there may have even been times that it was necessary to lift 100 pounds or greater. However, lifting 300 pounds on a weekly basis was not likely to occur. Although these types of exercises can lead to great results physically in the short term, there is a cost. Many of the guys and gals you see in the gym putting up extreme amounts of weights will eventually suffer an injury that could have the potential to impact them for the rest of their lives.

Now that you are looking through the lens of intended design, I hope you are starting to see why certain things make sense and certain things don't. Walking, running shorter distances, and working out with body weight fits the formula of human design. Hopefully you are also starting to see that exercise was not meant to help you lose weight, our ancestors didn't have that problem. Exercise stimulates the nervous system to help boost your immune function, increase your energy level, and relieve stress. Once you began exercising for the right reasons and the right way, you are more likely to stick with it.

Chapter 3: DIET

Similar to exercise, there is a lot of misinformation surrounding diet. One article you read says that coffee is good for you, but another article says that caffeine is bad for you. Which article is correct? The answer is pretty simple. Yet again, if the caveman didn't consume it then it probably goes against nature's intention. And if it goes against nature's intention then it probably isn't good for you.

Personally I believe that the only liquid the human should consume on a regular basis is water, and lots of it. If you or anyone in your family is consuming soda or milk you are poisoning yourself. The major protein in milk, casein has been implicated in studies as the likely cause of cancer. The sugars in soda are also suspected in "feeding" cancerous cells. Milk and sugary drinks like soda are what I call liquid poisons.

Unfortunately we have been bombarded with advertisements and slogans like "Milk...it does a body good." This couldn't be further from the truth. Science is starting to reveal all of the hazards of consuming dairy products. Cardiovascular disease, cancer, and diabetes can all be linked to consumption of dairy.

Take it back to the days of the caveman. What do you think he drank? Water, water, and more water. Can you imagine a caveman attempting to drink milk? I doubt our ancestors ever attempted to crawl underneath a wild buffalo and sneak a few drops of milk. It's pretty funny to think about a caveman trying to drink milk directly from a wild bison, but it is a great way to emphasize how unnatural the concept of drinking another animal's milk is. Who among us would drink milk straight from a cow's udder? Disgusting! Yet somehow we find it acceptable to chug a glass of milk with our breakfast, against nature's design.

Infants and toddlers have a special enzyme that they produce to process their mother's breast milk, but that enzyme disappears as they enter into adolescence. Again we see that nature intended for babies to drink their mother's milk but not other animals…and especially not into adulthood! Did the early homo sapien breastfeed? Certainly! It is natural and the perfect design for the growing baby.

I already can imagine what some people are thinking…cow's milk has protein and it's good for you. Yes, cow's milk does have lots of protein. It has the perfect amount for a baby cow, but way too much for a baby human, or even an adult. As a society we eat way too much protein, which has negative affects on our health. Take the Atkins diet as an example. It disappeared for a number of years because it was killing people…literally. The volume of protein was ripping tiny holes in the kidneys of people on the diet. It later reemerged with a higher water intake requirement to attempt to compensate for the harmful effects of excessive protein intake. This will be addressed later in the chapter.

Soda…the other liquid poison that is slowly killing our society. Unlike milk, soda has absolutely no nutritional value whatsoever. There is never a reason to drink a soda…ever. One of the root causes of disease in America, in my opinion, is sugar consumption. Studies have shown that eating sugar has the same effect on the brain as cocaine. Why would you expose your child to this product?

As a society we frown upon alcohol and marijuana as gateway drugs, yet we stuff our kids with sugar on every special occasion. Then we wonder why we are seeing a rise in ADHD. As this book is being written, 12% of American children are currently diagnosed with ADHD. It is becoming an epidemic. Looking at the data from the CDC website, the rise in ADHD coincides with the invention of high fructose corn syrup. I propose that sugar consumption is the main proponent of this disorder. And that is just one negative effect.

Obesity, diabetes, cancer, and cardiovascular disease all relate to sugar intake, particularly soda. I can't think of a good reason to ever give a child a sugary drink like a soda. Whenever I have this discussion with parents the argument is often the same, "We only drink soda on special occasions and we rarely buy it to keep in our home." The problem here is that there is a special occasion almost every weekend. Between birthday parties, sporting events, and holidays there is always a reason to celebrate. If you give your kids soda you are exposing them to the real American gateway drug…sugar. I take a hard-lined approach with soda, as there is no nutritional value and numerous reasons to avoid it. My children know that they are only allowed to drink water and they live full, happy, healthy lives. They can focus in school, play all day without running out of breath, and they rarely get sick. I see no reason a child should ever be given a soda.

Water, on the other hand, receives the physiological stamp of approval. Every morning when I wake I drink a full glass of water. At night before I go to sleep, again I drink a full glass of water, and throughout the day I drink water constantly. Dehydration is a huge problem in our culture and it can lead to many of the common conditions that we suffer from, including headaches and constipation.

As an aside, let me recommend another health tip. The next time you are suffering from a headache, instead of reaching for the Tylenol first, trying drinking water. In my estimation up to 80% of headaches are caused by dehydration alone. It is now very rare for me to get headaches, but when I do I start to chug glasses of water. Usually after 1-2 glasses the headache will start to subside. On occasion I will have to drink 4-5 glasses before it goes away, and on very rare occasions the headache won't go away, so I just go to sleep and it is gone by the time I wake up. Warning-side effects of this method include needing to use the restroom!

Now let's take a look at the concept of dieting as a whole. It always seems goofy to me when people talk about going on a diet. By definition, a diet is a temporary change. Yet people act surprised when a diet doesn't yield permanent results. I have news for you: if you want permanent results you will have to make permanent change. Don't go on a diet, change your eating habits. That is the only way to get results that last.

I recommend doing things slowly to give your physical and mental body a chance to adapt to the change and increase your chance for success. I think another reason so many people fail when they try to make changes is they try to do too much too quickly. Although I am not going to take the time to tell you exactly what to eat, when to eat it, etc., I will provide some simple steps and general guidelines to help you start your journey.

Step 1-Eliminate liquid toxins like soda, sweet tea, and coffee with a bunch of sugar in it. If you have to have coffee in the morning or tea, I understand. I have been able to eliminate sugar in my coffee and I take it with almond milk instead of dairy. Once you have eliminated these sugary drinks and replaced them with water you will feel a lot better. The pounds will slowly start to disappear just with this one change. Keep in mind that I said slowly. This is not a "lose-weight fast" scheme. Just sound advice on how to make permanent change. Drink a full glass of water first thing in the morning, one before each meal, and one right before you go to bed at night. Your body will be better hydrated and will thank you for it.

Step 2-Eat a salad for lunch Monday-Friday. You can have meat on it like chicken, shrimp, or beef. The main point of this step is to start to replace unhealthy dietary choices. Another hallmark of the standard American diet is lack of green leafy vegetables. Eating a salad each day will start to infuse your body with the nutrients that it needs to perform optimally, and you will also notice after a few weeks that your taste buds will change. You will actually start to crave a salad on the weekends too! I know because this is exactly what happened to me.

Step 3-Start replacing processed foods with natural products like fruits, vegetables, nuts and seeds. I would recommend packing a snack bag for yourself. Put whatever you like in your bag, but make sure it isn't processed. Typically I pack myself a banana or two, and apple, an avocado (to throw on my salad), and a sandwich baggie full of trail mix. The trail mix is clutch on those days that you get really hungry! Between the salad for lunch and your fresh fruit snacks, you are well on your way to an optimal diet!

Step 4-start limiting your intake of animal proteins. As I mentioned before, I try to limit my consumption of meat as much as possible. I do eat eggs and fish on a regular basis, but I avoid pork, chicken, and beef for the most part. During my studies I began to see a pattern emerge from a wide variety of materials that all pointed to the same thing-animal products like beef, chicken, and pork cause inflammation. I started thinking about how the caveman lived and it made sense to me that fish and eggs were consumed heavily. Think about it...early man always lived near a water supply, so fish were abundant and easy to catch. Eggs were also likely easy to come by near the water as many types of fowl nest there. I am sure the caveman ate meat as well, but I doubt that it was anywhere near the rate that we consume it today. I imagine that the major part of the caveman diet came from food that could be foraged: nuts, berries, fruits, roots, and even bugs.

These are the steps that I have taken to improve my diet, and it has helped me enjoy optimal health. I very rarely get sick, my allergies have disappeared, I almost never get headaches, and I maintain a healthy weight with very little effort. In the beginning it wasn't easy, but once my new healthy choices became habits I no longer needed to think about them. Eating a salad for lunch just became what I did every day. I can eat a lot because I eat the right foods and my body has grown to crave this type of diet. Counting calories is too complicated and that leads to failure. Take a page from the caveman playbook and eat tons of fruits and vegetables. No need to keep up with calories or weigh your food-it's all you can eat!

I often hear people say, "I could never eat like that. I like meat too much." First of all, and I am a firm believer in this concept-what one person can do another can do. You CAN do it, you just don't want to at this time. Most of us wait until there is some sort of serious health event before we make a change. It took a diagnosis of diverticulitis to open my eyes. Luckily that was not a serious condition and it disappeared immediately after I started eating right. Secondly, don't underestimate the body's ability to adapt to your new routine. As I mentioned before, I began to crave salads on the weekends after only a couple of weeks of eating one for lunch. On very rare occasions I will get a hankering for a steak or some bacon…so I have some! The key to successful dieting is not to diet at all, but to make permanent changes. You don't have to be crazy about it, just stick to the plan above and realize that it took years for you to get to where you are today, so logically it will take years to reverse any damage you have done to your body. At the time that I am writing this book, my journey towards optimal health has been over ten years in the making.

Chapter 4: POSITIVE THINKING

In my opinion this area of health is the most understudied, underestimated, and most revolutionary of all the topics that will be discussed in this book. The beginning of your journey into optimal health starts in your mind, as do all things. If you take radical steps to improve your wellbeing but ignore your mental state, I doubt you will be as successful as you hope to be. Let me give you an example of how negative thinking can stop the healing process before it even begins.

Early on in my time at Parker University, a friend contacted me seeking help. This old buddy had developed advanced osteoarthritis, a degenerative disease in his spine that normally is not seen until people are over 60 years of age. Unfortunately this early onset was attributed to weight gain, which was adding years of stress to his spine.

As you can imagine he was distraught over the pain, but also the prognosis given to him by the medical doctors. The only real solution given to him was to lose weight. At the time I had not studied osteoarthritis yet, so I took some time to research the condition, talk to my professors about it, and finally I concluded that the medical doctors were correct with the caveat that chiropractic care can also help to reverse the degenerative process.

Fortunately my friend was already under chiropractic care, so there was hope! After I was satisfied that I had done my due diligence in researching the condition I called him up to offer my services as a health coach, which he gladly accepted. "Ok!" I said, "Let's get started! The first step is to eliminate liquid toxins like sugary drinks, soda, sweet tea, etc." There was a long pause and he finally said, "Ahhhh…I'm not sure I can give up sweet tea." My response was to the point, "This is the first step in losing weight, so when you are ready give me a call."

I'm sorry to report that I have never heard back from my buddy on his attempting to lose weight. We remain friends to this day, but we don't discuss health issues. I figure that he will walk through that door when he is ready, and it is not my job to pressure anyone into changing his or her lifestyle. My job is to educate and to make people aware of the incredible option that is optimal living!

The point of the story is to show how so many people suffer from the "I could never do that" syndrome. As a vegetarian I hear that phrase all the time. "Oh you're a vegetarian? I know it's really healthy but I could never give up bacon." I always smile and say, "I understand, bacon is delicious." The thing people don't realize is that salads are delicious too, once you give your body a chance to fall in love with the flavor.

What one person can do, another can do. I firmly believe in this statement and I live my life by it. That is the positive mindset that is required to get any change started. We are all different and special in our own ways, but I don't think anyone deserves to be put on a pedestal here on earth. Should you admire people? Yes! Should you emulate positive habits of others? Yes! That being said, I think you should realize that the people you look up to are just that...people. The qualities you admire most in them are things that they had to WORK at, I guarantee it.

Many of the successful people that I have encountered have shared the secret to their success. Hard work, practice, and a positive attitude. Can you imagine someone being super-successful without believing in themselves first? Often times what we recognize as genius is the culmination of a lifetime of failures. Consider that.

Every action begins as a thought, and that thought travels from the brain down the spinal cord to every cell, tissue, and organ in the body. This is why it is so important to get your thought process straight first and foremost. Your mind can even affect hormonal levels!

Before you embark on any change, I want you to see yourself enjoying the new life that you chose. Next go beyond seeing and spend some time feeling. Imagine how you are going to feel in your new improved body. You can call it meditation, visualization, whatever you like. The end result should be the same-preparing your mind for change.

I am confident change would have occurred if my friend had said, "I can imagine myself drinking water, losing weight, living a life free of back pain." Anything is possible, but it has to start in your central command center, your brain. Nobody can put the thoughts in your head except you.

Every day I spend time visualizing my ideal self. My vision includes my children, my dream home, and of course my future self. I am in great shape, smiling, happy, and I am enjoying my life. To me it just makes sense that every possibility in your life begins with a vision. If you spend time focusing on this vision each day you won't be surprised when it starts to happen. *Breaking the Habit of Being Yourself*, by Dr. Joe Dispenza discusses visualization and meditation techniques, and it is a book I highly recommend.

I also spend time every day listening to positive affirmations. Another great book, *Talking to Yourself Is Not Crazy*, by Dr. Larry Markson, taught me the importance of daily positive affirmations. In his book he gives you three different affirmations. I couldn't decide which one I liked the best so I decided to use all three. Instead of reading them every day I recorded myself reading them aloud into the voice recorder on my phone. When I get to work I stay in my truck, lean the seat back, close my eyes and listen to myself speaking the positive affirmation aloud. It takes 4 minutes and 52 seconds, and I am certain this is the most valuable 5 minutes of my day. I can notice a marked difference on the days that I don't do my positive affirmation. I encourage you to try it for yourself and with your kids!

Chapter 5: NERVOUS SYSTEM SUPPLY

This is the most important chapter in this book, even more so than the previous chapter on positive thinking. Why? If your nervous system is compromised, even the most positive of thinking will not reach the rest of your body. The same goes for diet, exercise, sleep, and every other concept that relates to health. If the messages are not relaying back and forth from brain to body, and body to brain, it is all for nothing. You live your entire life through your nervous system, whether you realize it or not.

Enter chiropractic. Spinal misalignments (subluxation) can cause interference to the nervous system, which effects health. Sometimes subluxations are symptomatic, but often they are not. The chiropractor detects and corrects these misalignments using the chiropractic adjustment. The adjustment is like a "reset" button that gives the body a chance to adapt to the next stressor it encounters.

Most people think chiropractic is about back pain, but my personal experience goes much deeper and has revealed the true value of the adjustment. Since I made a commitment to getting checked for subluxation on a weekly basis, I have noticed a marked improvement in my health. Better sleep, more energy, and rarely getting sick top the list. I have also noticed that I am more in tune with my own body.

I wrote at the beginning of this book about my belief that you are your own best doctor. One of the benefits of regular chiropractic care is the reconnection that occurs between you and your body. When you are more in tune with how your body is functioning it can help you in your day-to-day life.

For example, I can be a bear when I am hungry, tired, or stressed. In the last few years, after getting reconnected on a regular basis, I feel like I am better able to recognize why I am feeling upset. Towards the end of the day when something rubs me the wrong way, I can quickly identify why I am reacting to whatever it is that has made me upset. In the past I might have let a little thing bother me for the rest of the day without realizing that I was just hungry or tired. Now I shrug my shoulders and smile, moving on and quite comfortable in my new reconnected self.

I have noticed similar changes in my family as well. As I began my journey into the world of chiropractic, I encouraged my loved ones to get checked for nervous system interference also. After about a year of care, something amazing happened to my father.

Dad is a world traveler, and he has been around the world many times over. Quite often upon returning from one of his globetrotting sessions he would be sick for at least a few days. Even more often he would return home with a tale of some weird stomach virus that he picked up on the trip that actually forced him to stay in the hotel for some portion of his vacation. Gradually this story began to change.

Recently dad went with a tour group to Vietnam. There were 30 people in the group, mostly consisting of people his age since they are retired and have more time to travel, with the exception of the tour guide who was 28 years old.

About a week into the tour, a terrible virus started making its way through the group. It was really bad; causing everyone that caught it to lie in bed for at least a couple of days to recover. The virus spread from person to person until it had infected every single person in the group except for two. Can you guess who the two people were that had immune systems strong enough to resist the virus? You got it! My dad (72 years old at the time) and the 28 year-old tour guide. There is no doubt in my mind that my dad was able to resist the virus because his immune system was functioning at a higher level. There is plenty of data that has proven the chiropractic adjustment improves immune function. Even more amazing is the fact that the tour guide was familiar with that environment, so his body could have already had an immune defense stored up for that particular virus. If that were the case, than my father would stand as the only person in the trip without previous exposure to fend off the attack!

While in school my classmates and I checked each other for subluxation on a daily basis. Not only did we need the practice, but we also knew that the stress of the program we were going through was likely to cause a weakened immune system. However, being adjusted by my peers wasn't always peaches and cream. There were several days throughout the program that I walked out of the adjusting labs with a raging headache. Towards the end of the program I was tired of getting adjusted so frequently and began to question whether it was doing more harm than good. By the end of the semester I was ready for a break from getting adjusted so frequently!

In between the fall and spring semester, we had an extended three-week break from classes. During one of the breaks, about a week into it, I began having trouble sleeping. Another week passed and I continued to toss and turn every night, the entire time wondering why I was having so much trouble. I chalked it up to the fact that I wasn't on a set schedule. Then I went to visit my chiropractor. You can probably guess how this story ends-I slept like a baby that night! In fact I slept for 19 hours straight! Improved sleep is just one of the many beneficial global affects that is commonly reported as a result of chiropractic care.

My father and I are not the only members of the family that have benefitted from chiropractic. My sister, my mother, and my kids have great testimonials to share as well. Aimee, my only sibling, is a high-school English teacher. She began suffering from migraines in her early twenties and had managed those terrible headaches using traditional means, i.e. medication. Often when she got a migraine she would be forced to leave work, lay in her bedroom with all of the lights off as even light aggravated her symptoms.

Early on in school I realized that migraines were one of the many conditions that have a plethora of studies and testimonials documenting the effectiveness of chiropractic care. I passed this information along to my sister, who was hesitant at first. I was sure that the adjustment could help her condition, so I went as far as to research chiropractors near her home. I found a doctor two blocks away who had a number of great reviews, so I called to talk to her. She was very nice, and when I told her about my sister's migraines she was confident that she could help.

After much persuasion, my sister started to see Dr. Phan. I am happy to report she saw a reduction of symptoms immediately! In the past she suffered migraine attacks on average twice a month. The first month into her care she reported that when she felt a headache coming on she would go and get adjusted, which would keep the headache from getting worse. Not only that, she told me that she really enjoyed her weekly visits to the chiropractor because it was one of the only times she felt that she got to relax. I was happy to have helped my sister connect with Dr. Phan!

One Saturday morning a few months later, my sister gave me a call. A very weak voice came through the phone, "Daniel, I have a migraine and Dr. Phan is closed. Can you come over and check me?" "Of course!" I replied. I packed up my portable adjusting table and drove to her house. When I arrived I was shocked to see her condition. She was lying down in her bed with the lights off, covered in a blanket with a scarf wrapped around her head. She was wearing sunglasses and could hardly walk down the stairs. When I say this woman was in pain I am not exaggerating. You can imagine the concern on the faces of my brother-in-law and two nephews as mommy was out of commission!

As she wobbled her way towards the adjusting table I noticed that she was very pale. I checked her neck and found a major subluxation at the second cervical vertebrae. I adjusted the segment and helped her up onto the couch. What happened next blew my mind! We sat on the couch and talked, and I could literally see the color returning to her face right before my eyes. Within five minutes she took off her sunglasses and commented how the light was not bothering her anymore. Another five minutes and she took off her scarf, as she didn't feel cold anymore. By the time I left she was back to normal, able to spend her valuable weekend time with her husband and two sons.

As an aside, I do not recommend using chiropractic as a band-aide or a method to treat conditions. You can choose to use it this way, but the real value of chiropractic is dependent upon regular care. Assuredly you will begin to feel better quickly, many people respond well to their first adjustment, but it would be in your best interest to make a commitment to get checked on a weekly or bi-weekly basis for at least a year. I understand that this can be quite a commitment in both time and money, but I am willing to wager that you will actually save both time and money by not missing work as often, not spending money or time in the medical doctor's office, and feeling this great, as I can attest, is priceless.

In conclusion and in accordance with the theme of this book, I must ask the question: Should chiropractic be considered a part of the intended design lens that you now look through? Absolutely! Your body was designed to stand up straight with your head perfectly balanced over your shoulders; your spine should have nice curves from front to back and be straight up and down. Subluxations, although naturally occurring, should be corrected immediately. Any interference to the signals between the brain and the body can have serious detrimental effects to your health.

Chapter 6: CHIROPRACTIC MIRACLE

During the first half of my education, I was lucky enough to work in a chiropractor's office, where I witnessed an amazing series of events. I hesitate to call it a "chiropractic miracle" because in reality, things like this happen in chiropractic clinics all the time. That being said, it is a miraculous story that I am going to share with you.

When Regina first entered Dr. James Bridges' clinic she was in a wheelchair. Unable to walk, talk, or feed herself, nine year-old Regina was teetering on the edge of a catatonic state. All that was about to change.

Three years ago Regina suffered an injury to her head and neck. Following the injury she began to have seizures and was diagnosed with epilepsy. She was given medication to keep the seizures under control, but unfortunately her body began to develop a tolerance to the medications and the seizures returned.

The cycle continued for the next three years. New larger doses of anti-seizure drugs were prescribed, which would hold off the seizures for a time, but eventually Regina's body would require more medication to keep the seizures at bay. Eventually she was on such a high dose that she was barely conscious and unable to function as a normal child.

Luckily a family member found Dr. Bridges. His unique approach to health care focuses on the nervous system, which accounts for his ability to discover issues that other doctors typically pass over. Regina's case was no exception.

After an initial exam Regina was found to have several misalignments in her cervical spine. According to Dr. Bridges, the trauma associated with her injury was the likely cause of this misalignment. Wasting no time, and with gentle pressure applied the treatment process began.

The first adjustment brought a miracle! Regina moved her right arm. Needless to say, her mother burst into tears. This was the first time in over a year that her little girl had made a voluntary movement. It wasn't much, but it was something different. A glimmer of hope appeared in what had been a very dark and cloudy three years.

Treatment continued for the first week, including house calls over the weekend to ensure that Regina held the adjustment. At the end of those first seven days Regina walked into the clinic on her own.

Now months into treatment Regina is walking, talking, feeding herself, and doing a lot of other things that normal nine year-olds do. When interviewed her mother says that the only thing they have done differently is began chiropractic care with Dr. Bridges.

Chapter 7: INNATE INTELLIGENCE

WE CHIROPRACTORS work with the subtle substance of the soul. We release the prisoned impulse, the tiny rivulet of force that emanates from the mind and flows over the nerves to the cells and stirs them into life.

We deal with the magic power that transforms common food into living, loving, thinking clay; that robes the earth with beauty, and hues and scents the flowers with the glory of the air.

In the dim, dark, distant long ago, when the sun first bowed to the morning star, this power spoke and there was life; it quickened the slime of the sea and the dust of the earth and drove the cell to union with its fellows in countless living forms.

Through eons of time it finned the fish and winged the bird and fanged the beast. Endlessly it worked, evolving its forms until it produced the crowning glory of them all.

With tireless energy it blows the bubble of each individual life and then silently, relentlessly dissolves the form, and absorbs the spirit into itself again.

And yet you ask, "Can Chiropractic cure appendicitis or the 'flu'?"

Have you more faith in a knife or a spoonful of medicine than in the innate power that animates the internal living world?

~B.J. Palmer

I would be remiss if I discussed chiropractic without discussing Innate Intelligence-it's kind of a big deal! Although modern science has not been able to prove the existence of Innate Intelligence, I think most people agree that there is something inside of our mechanical bodies that amounts to more than just a sum of our parts.

How else could you explain the following occurrence? When people undergo organ transplants, they will often start to develop new habits, cravings, or inclinations towards very specific hobbies. When the families of the organ donors are interviewed, the habit, craving, or tendency is always something that they recognize from their loved one. In one case, a very straight-laced church going lady received a kidney from a donor who died in a motorcycle accident. Following the surgery, the lady began to develop cravings for fried chicken and oddly enough she began to suddenly enjoy loud rock and roll. Neither of these things had appealed to her before the surgery. The family of the donor was tracked downed and questioned, and low and behold, the donor's favorite thing to eat was-fried chicken! You probably won't be shocked to find out that he also enjoyed listening to his rock-and-roll as loud as possible. How is it that these desires were "transferred" to the person accepting the organ? In my opinion Innate Intelligence is the answer.

There is something very powerful inside of you, running your body at all hours of the day and night. You don't have to think about breathing, pumping your blood, or healing the cut on your finger-it just happens! Take a moment and reflect on the amazing intelligence that would be required to run such an operation. Just the logistics are staggering! I wonder if even the most technologically advanced super-computer could handle the vast amount of data that is required to maintain homeostasis in the human body. The good news is you don't need a super-computer...you ARE the super-computer!

The Innate Intelligence within you is on a mission, to constantly maintain organization in your body. And you should trust that intelligence! If there is one thing that I hope you take away from this book it is this concept: You are your own best doctor because you know more about your body than anyone on the outside ever will. We even have common phrases in our society that point to the power within. Trust your instincts. Go with your gut. Follow your intuition. All of these clichés are trying to get the same message across-YOU HAVE AN INCREDIBLE INTELLIGENCE INSIDE YOU...WHY NOT TRUST IT?

In concluding this chapter, I would like to again stress the true value of chiropractic. Chiropractors do not treat diseases or conditions. Instead, we detect and correct vertebral subluxation to allow your body to function properly. When vertebrae in your spine become subluxated it lessens the ability of Innate Intelligence to perform the daily chores that are necessary for you to survive, and that's a problem. Whether you are currently symptomatic or not, it is a good idea to make sure your body can function properly. Get in touch with a great chiropractor and get yourself adjusted on a regular basis.

Chapter 8: STRESS VS. TOXIC LOAD

One of the most confusing aspects of health these days is the sheer volume of information. Furthering the dismay is the fact that information sources often conflict with one another. Coffee is good for you because it is a mood stabilizer, but too much caffeine can lead to insomnia and stomach problems. Alcohol, especially red wine, has proven health benefits, but too much can lead to a myriad of health issues. Do you see where I am going with this?

Unfortunately, the lens of intended design would not approve of either coffee or alcohol. From the strictest, very black and white viewpoint, neither of these beverages was designed to be consumed by the human body. However, I personally believe that the harmful effects of both of these beverages, along with other stress-relieving activities can fall into the category of "healthy when used correctly".

Consider this: The Guinness Book of World Records lists Jeanne Louise Calment as the oldest person to have lived at 122 years 164 days at the time of her death. Born in France, Calmet drank a bottle of red wine with her dinner every night and smoked one cigarette. Do you find this counterintuitive? If there is a "secret ingredient" to health and longevity it is finding a way to relieve stress. Stress is the only cause of disease. Not germs, not genetics. The only time the body falls ill is when it is under a stress that it cannot adapt to. Find a way to get rid of stress by exercising, meditating, reading, having a glass of wine, whatever it takes to unwind. Even if that means smoking one cigarette every night I believe that the good outweighs the bad.

As long as the stress-relieving effects of the activity outweigh the toxic load that it puts on the body I would put it into the healthy category. The question then becomes-how do I know if I am reaching the point where the toxic load is exceeding the beneficial effects? This is where your Innate Intelligence becomes very valuable. When you are listening to your body it will give you subtle clues.

All things in moderation, it is really that simple. Everything can be dangerous when abused; even things that are generally considered healthy, like water or exercise. I remember watching a story on the news when I was 12 years old where a man died from drinking too much water. If I remember correctly he had drunk 2-3 gallons in one day after being stranded in the desert for a number of days. Yes, this is a rare instance, but it emphasizes the point quite well, things are not always so black and white where health is concerned.

Chapter 9: GENETICS

Genetics is a hot-button topic in informed circles these days, and the cutting edge of science points to an imminent paradigm shift in thinking. More and more biologists, doctors, and informed consumers are coming to realize that genetics play a limited supporting role in determining health. Unfortunately, huge shifts in understanding take years to become established by the general academic community, so genetics is still being taught in schools.

It is an attractive theory, genetics, in that it is something we can map and control. A linear approach to health, wouldn't that be great? This is the main reason that so much stock has been placed into genetics, the thought that we can identify genes that cause disease. If the human genome can be mapped and disease-causing genes identified than we can take steps to control or stop the diseases altogether right? How is that working out so far? We already know which genes "cause" breast cancer, yet it still affects thousands of women each year.

I am aware of a patient who had a double mastectomy after learning that she did indeed carry the dreaded breast cancer gene. She went on to develop cancer in other parts of her body, including liver and lung. This is the problem with putting your faith in genetics, it is misplaced trust.

Genes do not cause Cancer, so removing tissues from the body is not a good way to go about prevention, in my opinion. The majority of diseases, like cancer, can be contributed to environmental factors. The new train of thought is that genetics only account for 5% of health outcomes, yet millions of dollars are being poured into this type of research annually. Why? Because there is money to be made. If a so-called disease-causing gene can be identified, you can make money developing a drug or a procedure to specifically fight that gene. The market driven health care market that has developed in the past century is pushing our research dollars towards profitable, tangible procedures and medications…that turn a profit.

This is the wrong approach. If modern medicine were truly concerned with the health of the consumer, it would focus on epigenetics. Epigenetics is the study of how environmental factors affect genetics and in turn health factors. This lion's share (95%) of factors determining health should be the brunt of research, but there is a huge problem-there isn't a lot of money in prevention.

All of the intended design concepts are addressing environmental factors. Sleep, exercise, diet, nervous system supply, and positive thinking are all important components…and they all share a commonality in that they don't turn a 2000% profit as many medications do. So there is the crux of the matter. Epigenetics, environmental factors, and prevention take a back seat in the medical model because they are not profitable.

Do you need proof? Consider the following: In the United States, African Americans are considered high-risk for diabetes. This is generally attributed to genetic factors. This is confusing to me because the rate of diabetes in Africa is much lower. In fact there have been studies done on recent immigrants that shows how the instances of diabetes increases when they move from other countries to America. Can someone explain this to me please? Did their genes change on the plane ride from Africa to America? I was under the impression that significant genetic change takes thousands of years! The only reasonable explanation is that genetics do not predispose us to disease to the degree that is advertised by modern medicine. Instead, our daily habits create changes in our body that encourage the expression of health or disease.

You are not genetically pre-programmed to die. Think about that for a moment. This is the current mindset of genetics! You are born with a genetic predisposition that you cannot escape. Your only hope is drugs and surgery. FALSE! If you are interested in learning more about epigenetics I suggest reading *Biology of Belief*, by Bruce Lipton, PhD.

52

Chapter 10: THE GERM THEORY

How is it possible that people living in the same household don't always fall ill when someone in the family is sick? How can medical doctors and nurses work in hospitals and not be sick all the time? What about teachers working with little booger-pickers all day? If germs caused disease than wouldn't all of these people be sick?

In fact, germs don't cause disease, weakened immune systems do. That is the only plausible explanation. When someone in the family gets the flu, there is no doubt that everyone living in the household has been infected by the virus. The only question at that point is whether or not their immune systems can battle the virus effectively.

A year into my doctorate program, a very virulent strain of the flu was making its way across the country. It was all over the news being touted as an epidemic. The first year of the doctorate program was extremely demanding as I was learning the "new language" of advanced sciences. Needless to say my nose was in a book so often I was completely oblivious to what was going on in the real world. My daughter came home from school one Friday in the midst of the epidemic, and she said that there were only five kids in her class that day because everyone was out sick with the flu. That means that 80% of the kids in her class had not been able to fight off the virus. I asked her if she knew whether any of the kids that were sick had received the flu shot? She said that the teacher had actually mentioned how surprised she was that many of the kids that fell ill had received the flu shot, while 3/5 of the kids that didn't fall ill did not get the shot (including my daughter). I was not surprised that she didn't get sick; she gets adjusted every week, which boosts her immune system!

My dad was listening in on the conversation and he asked what percentage of my class had caught the flu. This is when the light bulb really went off in my head. When I thought about it, I could only recall 1-2 people being sick in the past month, out of a class of 70+ people! When compared to my daughter's class it was an overwhelming statistic. I could only come to the conclusion that I was witnessing the power of the chiropractic lifestyle, which trumps a flu shot any day of the week, without the potentially harmful side effects. Health comes from the inside out, not the other way around.

Conventional wisdom states that bacteria cause disease and should be eliminated. This mindset is evident by the overuse of antibiotics and antibacterial soap in our society. We have declared war on bacteria. The bacteria are beginning to fight back with antibiotic resistant strains like MSRA. I propose a shift in thinking, a peace treaty if you will.

Bacteria have been here longer than us. Much longer. The first eukaryotic cells appeared 1.8 billion years ago, around the time that oxygen was becoming plentiful in the atmosphere. Since then they have not only survived, but thrived. Just recently humankind has begun this egotistical approach of attempting to "fight" bacteria.

Bacteria do not cause disease. Weakened immune systems allow disease to take hold. I can take a swab with a q-tip right now on the side of your face and culture numerous "harmful" bacteria including S. aureus, S. epidermitis, etc. These bacteria are EVERYWHERE! So why aren't we all dying from sepsis, endocarditis, or meningitis? Because our immune systems are doing their jobs day in and day out.

We will never eliminate all of the bacteria from our lives. Nor should we. Every bacterium is there for a reason and serves a specific purpose, which we may or may not understand at this point. Waging war on bacteria is a loser's game and I refuse to participate. Throw away your antibacterial soap and reserve antibiotic use for serious emergencies only.

Probiotics, chiropractic care, and other preventative measures should be the focus of modern scientific research. We should strive to find ways to support beneficial bacteria and boost our immune system. Living in harmony with bacteria is the only winning approach for survival of our species. Boosting our immune systems through optimal nervous system function is the way to go. Let me explain how this relates to chiropractic.

Chiropractic care has been proven to boost immune function in multiple studies. Increased serum thiol levels, decreased antibiotic use, and decreased hospital visits have all been attributed to the cumulative preventative effect that long term chiropractic care has on people. How does this relate to bacteria, probiotics, etc.? Good question.

The nervous system is the master controller of all of the body's functions. The vagus nerve in particular has been shown to play a vital role in natural immunity. The chiropractic adjustment stimulates the vagus nerve! If your brain is able to send clear messages to your gastrointestinal tract the beneficial bacteria work hard and remain happy.

Now I'm not saying to never wash your hands again or to drink directly out of a stream. Sanitation is important. However, this war on bacteria has reached its tipping point and it is time to adopt an approach that is more reasonable and more sustainable. First and foremost make sure your nervous system is functioning properly; this will allow the beneficial bacteria to do their job. Secondly you should consider a daily probiotic to repopulate your gut with good flora. Last and not least eat plenty of whole foods, which good bacteria love!

Chapter 11: PLAY IN THE GARDEN

I am a huge fan of gardening, for many reasons. Exercise, sunlight, healthy food, and interacting with beneficial bacteria are all great reasons to start a garden. Not to mention the positive impact it has on the environment! We are facing a health crisis in the United States, and I believe gardening could be a very effective tool to battle this crisis.

To me gardening is the pinnacle of personal responsibility as it relates to health, there is no better feeling than growing and eating your own food. From start to finish you have worked like crazy to dig, plant, and water your plants. You have stimulated your mind by researching what to plant, how to plant, and when to plant. And then you get to enjoy all of your hard work with a juicy tomato or delicious salad!

In this increasingly fast-paced and disconnected society, gardening provides a chance for friendship and exchange. I have met some of the most amazing people through the gardening community. It is also a great way to bridge the gap between the young and the old. Many of my gardening mentors are from a different generation, but we share a love for growing our own food. I cherish the moments with these mentors and the knowledge that they have passed down is invaluable.

Imagine a neighborhood where nobody has grass in the front lawns, instead they all have vegetable gardens. Think of the possibilities that this could create! Instead of going inside and watching television, everyone would be outside working in their yards, talking to one another, trading food and seeds. Information would be exchanged and neighbors would once again get to know one another. It is completely possible to do this! I would love to live on a street where every house had a front yard garden!

Why the front yard and not the backyard? We are disconnected as a society, and this is one of the factors that is causing increasing rates of depression in all age groups. Let's start talking to each other again! Imagine the amazing health and knowledge the children growing up on that street would enjoy. The elderly people in the neighborhood would benefit as well; what can make you happier than interacting with young children?

How about the science to support gardening for health benefits? One of the main reasons to garden is vitamin D. As a population we are deficient in this critical vitamin as a whole. Your body is such an incredibly amazing, intelligent machine. When you go out in the garden and enjoy some sunlight your body knows just how much it needs, when you start to get a little red it is time to go inside! Vitamin D supplements are great, but nothing can compare to the power of the sun, and natural vitamin D gain is preferred.

Another incredible aspect of gardening is the exercise that you get from working outside. As any experienced gardener can tell you, it ain't easy! Digging, weeding, and planting all require you to bend, twist, push and pull. This is great news! Think back to the chapter on exercise and you will recall that our bodies are designed to move in a certain way. Gardening provides the opportunity for movement that is natural and the end product is delicious foods!

Many gardeners agree that the secret is in the soil. Usually they are referring to how a good, healthy soil is necessary to be a successful gardener. An important component of healthy soil is beneficial bacteria, which allows plants to thrive. Would you be surprised to discover that the same beneficial bacterium that helps plants is now being studied as an anti-depressant? When you get out and "play in the dirt" you are actually recolonizing your skin with healthy, beneficial bacteria that keep your body chemically balanced.

Let's review the benefits of gardening. Reconnecting to your neighbors and your natural environment, growing your own amazing organic vegetables and fruits, getting your necessary vitamin D, exercising, learning, discovering, and exposing yourself to beneficial bacteria. From a health care perspective, gardening may be the most beneficial self-guided activity to improve overall well being.

Chapter 12: LISTENING TO THE UNIVERSE

As you might have guessed by now, I read a lot and I attend a lot of seminars. At one of these seminars I met Dr. Lona Cook, an amazing chiropractor, speaker, and author. She currently practices in Wisconsin where she owns and operates two clinics. She was one of the speakers at the seminar I attended, and a story she told that day changed the way I look at life.

When she was trying to decide where to open up her practice, she was having trouble picking between two locations. She really favored one location over the other, but everything she tried to do with that location didn't seem to work out. She was having trouble finding the appropriate sized building, and when she did the people that owned it were difficult to reach. You get the idea, one thing after another. With her second choice, however, everything just seemed to fall into place. She quickly found the ideal sized office, and the realtor she was working with was expedient, friendly, and knowledgeable. But it was her second choice! How many of us would have fought, pushed, kicked, and screamed our way into the first office? That was Dr. Cook's first instinct, which is understandable. We are trained to fight, fight, fight. Never give up. A champion never quits, etc. But what if we are choosing the wrong battles? What if we are trying to force our way into a place we were never meant to exist? Luckily, Dr. Cook had a mentor that told her to "listen to the Universe". She did…and it changed her life. She decided to focus on her second choice and the magic began to happen. Without giving away the entire story, let's just say she became wildly successful in a very short time at the "second choice" location.

I started thinking about what she said, and it made me realize that I had spent much of my life trying to force things. Jobs, relationships, you name it. When I realized that you could quiet the mind and focus on what the Universe is trying to tell you, amazing things start to happen. Relationships improve, you become more honest with yourself and everyone around you, and you become detached from results and expectations.

Upon further consideration I came up with a scale of proficiency for Universe Listeners: beginner, intermediate, and advanced. Are you curious to know where you stand on this grading scale? It is simple to self-assess.

The beginner is disconnected from the Universe and does not take time to quiet their mind. They don't meditate or visualize themselves being successful. There are clues all around the beginning Universe listener but they never listen to them. The trademark of the beginner is to try the same method over and over and expect a different result. Attempts are repeatedly made to force a square peg into a round hole. I speak from experience, as I was a beginner not too long ago. Before reading Dr. Cook's book, *Just Tell Me Where to*

Start! I never considered that the Universe could whisper to you, leading you in the right direction if you are just willing to listen. Does this sound too mystical? Consider the following: as a society we even have well-known clichés to describe the people that don't listen to the clues the world is giving them. We call them "lost" or "misguided"; we comment that he/she is "going down the wrong path". We can all agree that there are infinite roads of possibilities in our lives, represented by choices, and we can all agree that there is a best option at any given fork in the road. I encourage you to open your mind to the possibility that there are subtle clues that can help you decide which direction to travel. You just have to listen.

A few years ago I met a friend who was into meditation. Like most people I thought that it was weird. Isn't meditation something that hippies and Buddhist monks do? She invited me to a session that she was hosting and I politely declined. Then the strangest thing happened, I couldn't go a day without running in to meditation in some form or fashion. If I were reading a book meditation would be mentioned. At seminars, lectures, and even in conversation it kept coming up. Finally I realized that this was the Universe whispering in my ear, "This is something you need to look into!" I had already decided that I would attend the next session my friend hosted when I saw the billboard. I was driving along the highway and there it was, as plain as day. MEDITATION SEMINAR was big and bold and staring me right in the face. I couldn't help but laugh and yell as I passed the sign, "I HEAR YOU LOUD AND CLEAR UNIVERSE! I WILL START TO MEDITATE!"

Such is the plight of the beginner. Repeated taps on the shoulder, signs, and clues may go unnoticed. Perhaps they are stuck in a relationship that they shouldn't be in, or working in a field that they are not fit for, but despite all of the results they plod on in the wrong direction. The good news is, it is easy to get started!

There are plenty of books, audio files, and even YouTube videos that can teach you how to meditate and visualize. Spend some time each day quieting your mind and tapping into the fabric of the Universe. This is the first step in reaching the intermediate level. The intermediate Universe listener is able to pick up on clues that lead them in the right direction after just one or two nudges. I knew I was an intermediate when I would hear something a second time and know that it was meant for me to head in that direction. Before I began to pay attention to the clues around me, I might hear a book, movie, or idea dozens of times before I looked into it. When I finally bought the book, watched the movie, or tried the new idea I always thought to myself, why did I wait this long? The next evolution was hearing something mentioned twice and realizing that it was time for me to investigate. Now when I hear a book mentioned more than once I get online and order it. The only down side is I have a stack of books that I have not been able to get to!

As of now I consider myself to be an intermediate Universe listener, but I aspire to become an expert. Not being one myself I can only postulate how they exist. The expert Universe listener doesn't need any clues or taps on the shoulder. Instead they seek out the direction that suits them best in the fabric of space, before it materializes in the physical world. We have common terms for these people as well; we call them those who "make things happen." There is a lot of truth in that statement. Instead of waiting around for someone or something to guide them in the right direction, these bold pioneers create their own reality and are admired by the rest of us.

Chapter 13: DIPSHIT

Most of the classrooms at Parker University have huge windows on either two or three sides. This allows for some spectacular views, especially on the second floor classrooms. It is nice to be able to look outside and catch a glimpse of nature in between lectures. In one case, this spectacular view taught me an invaluable life lesson. This is the story of a bird named Dipshit.

The sun had just peaked over the eastern horizon, which caused a warm influx of sunlight into our classroom. I was enjoying the warmth of it while listening to the professor lecture that morning. Suddenly I heard a tapping very close to me. I looked over and there was a male cardinal, a brilliant red color, tapping on the classroom window with his beak. I quickly surmised that the sunlight had caused a reflection, and this beautiful bird had confused his mirror image for a competitor infringing on his territory. He continued to attack the glass, knocking his beak into his perceived enemy. After the lecture a few of us gathered and laughed at the silly little bird. One student exclaimed, "What a dipshit!" And so the bird was named.

That afternoon I went to my truck, and whom did I see but Dipshit. He was attacking his reflection again, this time in the window of the car next to me. He looked a little worn down and his feathers were ruffled. I wondered if he had spent his entire day knocking his head against windows, attacking his imaginary enemies. I let out a big sigh as I looked around; it was such a gorgeous spring day! What a shame that Dipshit was so concerned about this perceived threat.

The days became weeks, the weeks became months, and the semester was coming to an end. Dipshit continued to guard his territory ferociously, attacking his reflection repeatedly and without regard for his own health and wellbeing. He had a particular inclination to show up in the middle of an exam-as if Pathology was not difficult enough! He began to look worse and worse as the end of the semester approached. He had lost weight and his feathers were now ruffled and mangled permanently. I felt sorry for the bird and thought to tape pieces of white paper up on all of the windows in our classroom, but then again, I couldn't go around taping pieces of paper on every car window too! The best I could do was to hope Dipshit would eventually realize that he was attacking himself.

Then it came to me, like a tiny lightning bolt between my ears-I was Dipshit. I had been Dipshit my entire life. How many times had I "attacked my reflection", in other words, how many times had I gotten upset over something that I could have let go? You see, in an instant I came to understand that EVERY PROBLEM I HAD EVER HAD IN MY LIFE I HAD CREATED MYSELF. I am going to repeat that statement because it changed my life and I have a feeling that it could change yours as well. Every problem I have ever had I created myself. In every instance, in every argument, in every situation I CHOSE HOW TO REACT.

You may be thinking, what the hell is this guy talking about? Let me explain. Every encounter with another person is a reflection of you. For example, let's say someone cuts you off on the highway. You immediately honk your horn and throw up your hands while yelling, "YOU'RE A FREAKING MORON!!!" Your sympathetic nervous system turns on, your adrenaline levels go through the roof, and your stress level skyrockets along with it. You might be thinking, hey, the other guy cut me off, it wasn't my fault! But wasn't it? Didn't you CHOOSE to get angry, yell, and honk your horn? Didn't you just attack your own reflection? What did any of that yelling and honking achieve?

What about the last argument you had with your spouse. Was the issue really important? Were you arguing over money? Was it so important that you are still mad about it today? I would imagine not. In reality there was probably something YOU could have done better when discussing it with your sweetheart. Isn't it always true that we can improve how we deliver our message to the ones we love? You see, by not taking care to guard the emotions of your loved ones, you have been attacking your own reflection all along.

I think about Dipshit often, especially when I am involved in some kind of argument or facing a difficult decision. What a magnificent creature he was meant to be. Can you imagine being a bird, with the ability to fly high above the city and swoop down into stream for a drink and a quick bath? What a beautiful opportunity that Dipshit wasted every day. He was not living like a bird anymore, but more like a man. Jealousy, anger, fear, and greed had consumed his being to the point of his detriment. How many of us are attacking our own reflections? How many of us are allowing our health to decline over issues that don't really even exist? How many of us are missing beautiful days, these moments that will never be recaptured, over things that are as silly as money?

As I continue down the path of self-improvement I strive not to be a Dipshit. In every encounter I now walk away wondering what I could have done better. Even if I know the other person was 100% wrong, I still walk away thinking HOW COULD I HAVE DONE BETTER? Could I have been more kind, more understanding, could I have been a better listener? Could I have been more patient, more sympathetic, could I have interjected my opinion at a better point in the conversation? My communication with others has improved markedly since I adopted this new mindset, and I would encourage you to consider doing the same. Good luck on your journey and remember-every day is a gift!

Chapter 14: LOSING FAITH IN MODERN MEDICINE

I hesitate to write this chapter because in all honesty, I have mixed feelings concerning the medical model. On one hand, I have a deep respect for the medical community and I am extremely grateful for the hard work and dedication that doctors, nurses, EMTs and others involved in healthcare exemplify. As far as emergency care is concerned, there is no doubt in my mind that our hospitals are second to none. That being said, my personal experiences in my adult life have led me to believe that there is a lot of room for improvement in the way we handle chronic disease, the birthing process, and how people are treated in general. It seems that common sense and being the doctor is sometimes abandoned in exchange for money.

One of the scariest moments of my life happened during the birth of my younger son. My wife wanted to have a natural birth. She tried to get through the labor but when the contractions started to intensify she decided to go with the epidural. I have never experienced the pains of labor (obviously) and it is not my intention to pass judgement. If you feel you need an epidural during labor it is your choice ladies and I support that decision. That being said, I would like to share this story with you so that you know the risk involved.

When the anesthesiologist came into the room I felt fine. The he pulled out the needle that he would be inserting into my wife's back. I am not going to lie-I almost fainted. He glanced over at me and asked if I was okay. I thought I was hiding it well, the fact that I was about to pass out, but I guess I wasn't! I made it through without losing consciousness and I though everything was fine and dandy. Mommy seemed relaxed now and it looked like a smooth birth was about to take place. Suddenly the bleeps on the heart rate monitor started to slow, and then they stopped altogether. I looked at my wife and she was turning blue. She had stopped breathing. "What is going on?" I screamed to the nurse, who luckily was in the room at the time. "She is having a reaction to the epidural," she replied. I could see that she was visible shaking. "What should I do?" I asked. "Just stay calm sir, I've got this," was the nurse's answer. With shaking hands she started punching in numbers into the computer and loaded up a needle with epinephrine. She injected the drug into the IV and almost instantaneously my wife's heart started beating again. She took in a deep breath of air with a gasp and her face went from blue, to pale white, to full of color within a matter of seconds. She opened her eyes and looked around, stunned. "What happened?" she asked. "You died." I replied. Probably not the best answer but it was all I could come up with. "That's what I thought," she said calmly, "I felt like I was dying." We held hands and put our heads together, shedding tears and thanking God that her life had been spared. She went on to deliver baby Davy just hours later, a perfectly healthy baby boy. I am happy to report Davy is happy and healthy and did not suffer any birth trauma even though his mom did in fact die during his birth. The point of the story is to exhibit my opinion that although modern medicine produces countless miracles, it also walks a fine line at times. If I could sum it up in one sentence without prejudice, I would say that at the very least there are times when the medical establishment is very cavalier with peoples' lives.

The next hospital visit for Davy came three years later, when he developed RSV (respiratory syncytial virus). I was out of town at the time he entered the hospital, but dropped everything and drove from Dallas to San Antonio to be there. When I arrived he was having trouble breathing, his oxygen was at 82 (that's bad as it should be closer to 100), and according to the doctors his veins were on the verge of collapsing. His eyes were red and he was crying, but he immediately perked up when he saw me. I analyzed his thoracic spine (mid-back) and found multiple restrictions. I adjusted what I found, right there on the hospital bed, and watched his oxygen normalize within five minutes. His breathing improved just as quickly and the nurses were amazed at how much he had improved in a matter of minutes. I wasn't surprised at all…that's chiropractic! Originally the doctors had predicted he would need to stay five days to recover fully, but after he stabilized they revised the prediction to three days, and in reality he was released after only two days.

We were not out of the woods yet as Davy was still on a powerful steroid, which was causing some very serious side effects. He had been up for 24 hours straight and the steroid was not allowing him to sleep. In fact he was getting so bad that we had to hold him down, he was trying to pull his own hair out and grabbing the skin on his chest and trying to rip it off. I was livid and immediately recognized it as a reaction to the drugs. I called the nurse in and asked her if she could do anything, she replied that this type of reaction was normal. WHAT?!? When she left the room I turned to my wife and let loose a string of explicatives. I couldn't accept the fact that a three year-old kid pulling his hair and grabbing his skin until it bled was considered "okay" by these healthcare workers. We literally had to take turns restraining him! I called the nurse back and asked if we could give him something to calm him down, to counteract the steroid. Usually I am the last guy that would ever support giving a child more medication, but I felt that this had reached an emergency status. She said she didn't think the doctor would be willing to prescribe any more medication and that we would have to wait until it wore off. I asked her if the doctor would be willing to administer children's Benadryl, or if she knew of any other common over-the-counter medication that could help my poor baby sleep. Her face lightened up and she said, "That's a really good idea. I don't think Benadryl would react to the steroid, let me call the doctor and ask him." Sure enough the doctor approved the Benadryl and the nurse came in to give Davy the medicine. He was asleep in twenty minutes and he slept for 18 hours straight! When he woke up he was calm, all of his levels were normal, and we were released later that day. I rarely advocate the use of medication for children, but in this case the risk was worth the reward.

Again, I would like to express my gratitude for the hospital staff and those that work in medicine. I truly believe that you save lives every day and I thank you for it. That being said, my experiences in the hospital and with the medical community have led me to believe that there is plenty of room for improvement. This is understandable as the human body is an incredibly complex machine! I am not a medical doctor, but common sense told me that a three year-old pulling his hair out is not normal and that something needed to be done. In the case of my ex-wife, I am still not sure what happened. Perhaps she was given too much anesthesia or perhaps she had a reaction to the proper dose. No explanation was offered and to be honest we were so focused on our new baby boy we never followed up with the hospital or thought to question what had happened until much later. One would think that there would have been some sort of documentation or report generated for such an incident…it makes me wonder how many of these types of things happen on a regular basis and go undocumented. If I get into an accident take me to the hospital, but I try to avoid the medical institutions as much as possible. I have lost faith in the medical model outside of emergency care.

Chapter 15: THE BIRTHING PROCESS

The previous chapter has set the stage for this next topic. I believe that the birthing process is the start of the slippery slope that is our current healthcare system. Again, I would propose that hospitals and doctors are putting money, speed, and efficiency above the welfare of the patients, in this case, babies. More and more hospitals are encouraging cesarean sections, or C-section as it is commonly abbreviated. It makes sense to the hospital and the doctor from a financial standpoint. C-sections can be scheduled and planned for. That way the guesswork is taken out of birth. Doctors don't like to be woken up at 2:30 in the morning to come and deliver a baby-think about it!

The problem is, C-sections are not natural and unless the procedure is an emergency-type of medical necessity you are gambling with the wellbeing of your newborn. There are multiple reasons the C-section is dangerous. First and foremost is the method of delivery putting pressure on the skull and the cervical (neck) part of the spine. Have you ever seen a C-section performed? I invite you to watch a YouTube video of a C-section before you consider allowing it to be done to yourself, your wife, or especially your child.

Conditions like ADHD, SIDS, and autism in children are rising at alarming rates. If you compare the statistics you see an interesting overlay between the simultaneous rise in C-section rates for the same time period. There are a growing number of healthcare providers that believe there is a link. As a chiropractor this makes perfect sense to me. I now understand how subluxations of the spine can grossly affect health, and if you have ever seen a C-section performed you can easily see how it stresses and misaligns the cervical spine. This subluxation of the first few vertebra in the neck puts pressure on the spinal cord of the newborn baby, and that is not only harmful, in some cases it is deadly. A group of newborns that died from SIDS were examined afterwards and gross subluxations of the first cervical vertebra (C1) were seen in all cases. Is it possible that torsion to the neck during the birthing process could be at least a contributing factor to disease? I believe the answer is yes. In fact, there is already a disease that is known to be caused by birth trauma, cerebral palsy. Most of these cases involve the use of forceps or vacuum-assisted births, similar to the approach that is used in a C-section delivery. It stands to reason that less serious birth trauma (if there is such a thing) may go undetected for years, putting just enough pressure on the cervical spine and the spinal cord to contribute to these childhood diseases.

What can be done? Simply and plainly, get your child to a chiropractor as soon after birth as possible, especially if you have had a C-section. Adjustments performed on babies are very light and gentle, many times using the pinkies and putting the same amount of pressure as it would take to move a dime across a table. The same way you take your baby to a doctor to check their height and weight checked, you should have your baby's spine checked as well. How can you help potentially prevent a C-section? Get adjusted throughout your pregnancy. I am friends with an amazing chiropractor here in Dallas, Dr. Autumn Gore, who works closely with Baylor hospital. In fact, she is frequently invited to go into the hospital and adjust mommas during labor and babies immediately after birth. Since she began working in Baylor 7 years ago, C-section rates have fallen from 37% to less than 20%. That's amazing! If you are expecting get yourself to a chiropractor! If you have kids and they have never had their spine evaluated-what are you waiting for?

Chapter 16: CLEANSING

Getting back to the lens of intended design, it makes sense to me that physiologically we were made to go through periods without eating much. I love food as much as the next person, but it stands to reason that it may be healthy to reduce food intake periodically. Think of it as giving the digestive system a break, time to rest and regenerate. We can go for up to 30 days without eating, although this in not recommended it does point to the fact that we are designed to be able to withstand long periods without food.

Personally I have never gone more than a couple of days without eating, but I have tried different cleanses with good results. At this time I am on a cleanse, so this information is up-to-date and relevant! I am always experimenting (with myself) in an attempt to improve my own health. I will share my experiences with you and let you decide if it is something you may be interested in.

Currently I am trying a hybrid juice/low calorie intake cleanse. Basically I drink a cup of bulletproof coffee (coffee, butter, coconut oil) in the morning, drink fruit/veggie juice throughout the day, and I have a normal dinner in the evening. The goal of this type of cleanse is to give my digestive system a lighter load to work with and facilitate quick transit time. I have been encountering an increasing volume of literature that shows reducing caloric intake is really good for you. In other words, eat less and live healthier!

As you know, the American diet is out of control. Not only do we eat too much, the food we do eat is often not very good for us. I encourage you to take a break from what you normally eat, even if it is for only a few days. Try a cleanse a couple of times a year and give your digestive organs a chance to regenerate. The movie *Fat, Sick, and Nearly Dead* is a great resource for the juice cleanse. This movie is what really got me motivated to start experimenting with cleansing-without spoiling it for you let's just say the results are amazing! It is on Netflix and I highly recommend watching it.

Try a juice cleanse over a long weekend, so you are only on the hook for three days. It is really not too complicated, all you need is a whole bunch of fruits and veggies and a juicer. You will be surprised at how quickly your body adapts to the change. My recommendation is to drink plenty of water as you juice, one glass of water for every glass of juice you drink. You are going to be going to the bathroom often, but that is the point! You want to allow the body an opportunity to flush itself out.

If you don't think you can manage only drinking juice for two or three days, try a hybrid juice cleanse like I am. Do what you feel comfortable doing, remember-you are your best doctor! Try juicing for breakfast for a week and see how you feel. If you like it than perhaps you can go forward from there or at least add a breakfast juice into your daily routine.

Another type of cleanse that I highly recommend is Dr. Tim O'Shea's 60-day program and the New West Diet. I have personally tried this cleanse and the results were amazing. Go to www.thedoctorwithin.com for complete information. If you are a health-seeker like me, you will really enjoy his website.

The 60-day program is a serious cleanse and may not be the right choice for you unless you are willing to make some serious lifestyle changes, but I can tell you with 100% certainty it works. You will move toxins out of your system at an incredible rate as I can attest to. About a week into the 60-day program, on a Saturday morning, I started going to the bathroom. I now call that day "poop-fest". I woke up early even though it was a Saturday, around 6:45 if I remember correctly. Without giving you all of the intimate details, I used the restroom 5 times by 9:00 that morning. And I am not talking about little baby poops here; all 5 were king-kong sized dookies. Now most of you are probably thinking-ewwwww! Gross right? Well, it was a sign that things were shaking loose and moving out from my system. The only other option is that all of that waste sits inside my intestines and rot. When you see someone with a huge "beer belly" what do you think causes that? It isn't beer sitting in there and it is not all belly fat. In fact, the majority of people's gut is fecal matter backed up in their intestines. In other words, they are full of it!

My bathroom habits normalized after that one morning, and the next week something even more incredible occurred. I began to develop a rash on the back of my hands. I woke up in the middle of the night and my hands felt a little weird. I went to the bathroom and found a puddle of grease on the back of my hands, where the rash was. I got a towel and wiped it off, confused and amazed at the same time. I got on my computer and emailed Dr. O'Shea immediately, I was worried I was having some sort of reaction to the cleansing process. It didn't hurt or anything but it sure was out of the ordinary! I settled down to get some sleep and when I woke up the next morning Dr. O'Shea had replied to my email. He explained that the body naturally pushes toxins as far away from the important organs (brain, heart, lungs) as possible. The tissues in the hands and the feet, being the farthest away from the crucial, centrally located organs, are common places for the body to store toxins as a protection mechanism. The cleanse had encouraged my body to open up the pores in my hands and push out the toxins! After that night the rash started to clear up and went away all together within a few days. I completed the cleanse and felt amazing!

Chapter 17: VACCINATIONS

Vaccination is a hot topic right now. The pro-vax camp and the anti-vax camp have pitted themselves against each other and each side is dug in deep. I have remained open-minded and tried to avoid arguing with people about the subject because I have found that it is a very emotional subject, and understandable so. Parents with vaccine-injured children have a right to be upset and express their opinion. Parents of children who chose to vaccinate are worried that unvaccinated children put their child at risk, which doesn't make much sense to me but they have a right to express their opinion as well.

Herd immunity is commonly the rally cry of the pro-vax camp. There is a belief that if enough of the population is vaccinated against a disease that it will provide protection to the entire population. My first question is: if you were vaccinated why would you need to worry about it? The argument is that herd immunity protects the immune compromised individuals like newborns and the elderly. I would argue that bolstering the immune system with natural means should be the preferred method of presenting disease, for example breastfeeding in newborns and a preventative regimen for the elderly that includes diet, exercise, and of course chiropractic care for both populations. If you recall the story about my father when he traveled to Vietnam, you can see that this is the approach we take in my family, and I have seen the results.

One important point that I would like to make is that both sides have based their decisions on theories. There have not been any conclusive studies done on the efficacy of vaccines or the safety of the vaccines. The anti-vax camp has proposed a theory that the rise and fall of infectious diseases like polio, smallpox, and measles was a natural progression. It actually makes a lot of sense when you think about it. In the days of our early ancestors, the population was spread out and people went to the bathroom out in the woods and went on their way, so the disease associated with sewage and people crowding into a small space was non-existent. Think about the bubonic plague that killed millions in the middle Ages. The carrier for the disease was the flea, which traveled via rats. This was not a problem in the era of the caveman. Then we entered a time when populations came to live together and a migration towards the cities. This was the Industrial Revolution, and interestingly the rise of these diseases coordinates with the rise in population in the cities. In fact, you can take a line graph of the rise in population of city-dwellers during the Industrial Revolution and overlay a graph of the rise of disease and they will match very closely. The second part of the story is the fall of disease. The anti-vax camp postulates that diseases began to disappear because of improvements in drinking water, sewage treatment, and other factors that affect sanitary conditions. Again, historically this makes sense. The improvements in public sanitation following World War II coincide with the fall of common diseases that had previously plagued our society since the Industrial Revolution.

So the question remains-who is correct? Do vaccines prevent disease? In all honesty I have not seen any research that proves their efficacy, although I will admit the theory behind vaccines makes sense as well. Put a small amount of a virus into the body and allow an immune response to occur. The next time the body encounters the virus it will have stored antibodies to combat the virus. The theory makes, sense, but much like the anti-vax theory, it is just a theory. It has never been proven. There has never been a randomized controlled trial that compares the rates of disease between vaccinated and non-vaccinated individuals, so at this point I choose to trust my instincts, and you can probably guess the direction that has led me.

Is vaccine injury real? Yes. There is no doubt in my mind that vaccine injuries have occurred. In this matter there is research that is statistically sound, and it shows that neurological disorders, in many cases, can be attributed to vaccine reactions. There is also a special court that deals with vaccine cases. You can look it up online and read for yourself. The risk of vaccine injury is real and has been documented. The movie *Bought*, by director Jeff Hays discusses this topic and it is very well done. If you are interested in learning more I encourage you to check out this film.

Another option you may consider for your family is a reduced schedule. If you look at the vaccine schedule from the 1980s until present day, the number of vaccinations recommended has increased astronomically, yet the projected lifespan has decreased. I am not insinuating the two are necessarily related, but it is something to consider. Are the pharmaceutical companies interested in increasing health or increasing their bank accounts? That is a question that must be asked. If you believe in the validity of vaccinations at least take a look at which vaccines are necessary and which may be included in the increased schedule for profit.

For example, let's look at the Hepatitis B vaccine. It is part of the mandatory schedule for newborns, but Hepatitis B is contracted in two ways-drug use (sharing needles) or sexual intercourse. Why would a newborn need a vaccine for a disease like Hepatitis B? Why would you stress the immune system of a perfect newborn baby unnecessarily? In my opinion, taking your time to research the need for every vaccine is very important. If your pediatrician is not willing to discuss a reduced schedule for vaccination I would find a new doctor.

There is nothing in this book that I have not lived by. My own children received their first round of vaccines but I have stopped allowing further shots and chose instead to focus on bolstering their immunity with natural means. In retrospect I wish I had at least waited until their immune system had fully developed before I considered allowing any vaccinations; I feel like I dodged a bullet there.

Chapter 18: EMBRACING SYMPTOMS

A fever, a headache, or diarrhea is no fun. Many of us reach for a Tylenol, Pepto Bismol, or some other form of pain relief when we are suffering from one of these symptoms, and they do tend to make us feel better. But are we making the right choice?

Symptoms like fever, headache, and diarrhea are the body's way of expressing exactly what it needs to express at that moment. I think we can all agree that our body has an Innate Intelligence that is far superior to the intelligence of modern science; in other words, our body knows exactly what needs to be done to heal.

Fever, for example, is the body's defense mechanism to deal with viruses and harmful bacteria. Most harmful bacteria and viruses are classified as mesophiles, which prefer temperatures around 37 degrees Celsius, the normal temperature of the human body. When the body detects one of these invaders it cranks up the heat to kill the virus or bacteria, so why would we want to stop this process? Very high fevers, above 105 degrees Fahrenheit can cause neurological problems, but these types of fevers are very rare. It is completely normal to run a fever of 102-103 degrees in order for the body to rid itself of any foreign invaders.

Headache is another symptom that should be embraced, not suppressed. A headache can be an early warning sign to a myriad of issues. Many times headaches are related to dehydration, lack of sleep, or stress. This is our body's way of telling us that we need to take better care of ourselves. Taking a Tylenol or Advil makes you feel better and allows you to continue to pound away at the body, but in the end you are doing further damage.

Diarrhea is probably not the subject you want to discuss at a dinner party, but we have all experienced it at one time or another. It can be stress related, but many times this is our body's method for expelling foreign invaders (at times violently). Again, I must question why anyone would want to slow this process down? When you take Pepto Bismol or some other anti-diarrhea medicine you are effectively keeping these harmful invaders in your body longer, which gives an increased opportunity for infection. The "flood gates" are open for a reason, why would you want to shut them?

Practicing what I preach...my daughter complained of a stomachache this weekend on Saturday night. I had her drink some water and put her to bed, hoping that she would wake up feeling better. When I woke her up Sunday morning to start getting ready for church she said her stomach still hurt. I told her that we would stay home and to go back to sleep. She ended up sleeping until noon! But when she woke up, she felt great! The stomachache was completely gone. I could have given her Pepto Bismol or something to make her feel better, but I would have risked interfering with the body's normal function. Why would I do that? I have more confidence in the Innate Intelligence of the human body than the wisdom of the chemists who created Pepto.

All of these symptoms fall into the early warning sign category. Similar to the check engine light on your dashboard-fevers, headaches, and diarrhea can be indicative of more serious dysfunction if they persist. I would encourage you to seek out a healthcare provider that seeks out a cause for these symptoms and addresses the underlying stressor that is triggering the response.

Chapter 19-IDIOPATHIC DISEASE

Idiopathic disease is defined as a disease that does not have a known cause. You would be shocked to find out how many diseases are classified as idiopathic. I have never seen a figure put to it but I would guess the number to be at least 25% and possibly upwards of 50%. The point is we really don't know much about disease. Yes, as modern science improves we are learning, but we still have a long way to go.

When I entered the chiropractic college at Parker University I was excited to learn all of the things I would need to know to become an amazing doctor, in fact I still aspire to this day to become one of the world's greatest healers. My expectation was to have some incredible life-changing revelation, and I did! But it wasn't the mind-shifting change that I thought it would be. Instead it was a confirmation of what I already suspected.

I came into school healthy, with a good idea of what defined it. I believed before my education that diet, sleep, exercise, and a fully functioning nervous system were the keys to health. Exiting school I have realized that I was right...with the addition of positive thinking to aid in optimal health. This has been a novel concept.

Working at the Research Institute at Parker University provided me with the opportunity to read a great volume of scientific literature, including case studies, meta-analysis, and randomized controlled trials. In reading study after study patterns began to emerge. Obesity is the most accurate predictor of most disease. Lifestyle habits like caloric intake (how much you eat) and exercise were the only viable predictor of survival rates after a serious disease formed, for example ovarian cancer.

Although diseases like cancer and autoimmune conditions like rheumatoid arthritis are classified as idiopathic, in my mind the causes are clear. Lifestyle choices are the cause in most cases. There are exceptions, for example children who suffer from cancer. It is doubtful that this type of disease process could be attributed to a lifestyle choice. More than likely there is some sort of structural pathology that science has not yet been able to detect. But I digress. The classification of idiopathic disease, like genetics, has given people an excuse to separate themselves from personal responsibility.

I am not quite sure why modern medicine hesitates to attribute diseases to lifestyle choices. The ball is moving in that direction but ever so slowly. Epidemiological studies have proven how diet and other lifestyle factors contribute to disease. Historically their peers shun the doctors that speak out about this, perhaps that is the reason it is taking so long for the truth to emerge.

Lastly…what would it hurt to try to improve your health in the ways I have described? If you have an autoimmune condition, cancer, or any other idiopathic disease why not try to eat, sleep, move, and think well? Why not get your nervous system checked for subluxation? Why not improve all of the key areas of health? The worst thing that can happen is that you will become a health-nut, and that isn't such a bad thing.

Chapter 20: RCT vs. EPIDEMIOLOGICAL STUDIES, CASE STUDIES

The randomized control trial, or RCT is heralded in modern science as the "gold standard" of research. The theory is that eliminating as many variables as possible is the way to find the most accurate information. The RCT has at least two groups- a control group and an experimental group. The control group does not receive the treatment and the experimental group does. At the end of the trial the results are compared. The participants are a very narrow sample of the population, as narrow as possible. For example, a group of 100 men between ages 40-45 with similar health histories. The idea is that a group of people that are very similar to one another will give an accurate picture of the effect of whatever is being studied.

In comparison, the epidemiological study is considered less reliable because it does not have a control group. This type of study does not necessarily eliminate people based on age, health history, etc. Instead of trying to eliminate as many variables as possible, it accepts all variables and focuses on the thing being tested, whether it is a drug, food, or form of treatment.

Case studies are ranked as one of the lowest forms of scientific data. A case study is a write-up of one health outcome, for example, how a child diagnosed with ADHD underwent chiropractic care improved their ability to focus. The scientific community views this as "low-level" because it is only one person and according to conventional wisdom, it could be a fluke. But what about 5 case studies that observe similar results? What about 10? 20? 50? At what point do you recognize the value in this observation?

Another question I have-which type of study more accurately accounts for the human experience? Would you rather take a drug that was tested on a very small slice of the human race or would you prefer that a wide variety of the population were tested? Which do you imagine would offer you more protection?

The human race is full of diversity, and people will react differently to treatments. Instead of trying to eliminate variables, why not embrace them? We should be accounting for the variety of existence within our race when we go to study it. Just think of all the factors that can never be controlled.

Going back to our example, consider a group of men 40-45 with similar health histories. We put them in a group that we call "similar" but what about their diet? That alone could be one of the most important factors in how their bodies differ from a physiological perspective. Did you know there are 10,000 different chemical compounds in an apple? What about their sleeping patterns, love life, work situation, etc.? All of these are part of the human experience and it goes to show that eliminating variables is a false premise. Impossible to truly achieve.

Instead why don't we flip the hierarchy of reliability, placing a volume of case studies at the top and RCT's at the bottom? This more accurately reflects the human experience, in my opinion. Just one more thing-if drugs are approved via RCT, and that is the gold standard in research, how is it that drugs end up killing people and having to be recalled? If RCT's were truly reliable this would not occur.

Chapter 21: PILL POPPING

I grew up in the era when modern medicine was worshipped and trusted completely. If I ran a fever we ran to the drugstore. If the fever persisted we ran to the doctor. The doctor prescribed antibiotics and the cycle continued.

I never thought to question this method of treatment-it is the standard mode of thinking. You feel bad, go to the doctor and they will give you something to make you feel better. Isn't that basically what we do?

Unfortunately I think this sends the wrong message to children. We are unknowingly training them to seek "feeling good" from drugs. Is it any wonder we have problems in our society with addiction?

What if the next time you or your child has a fever you let the body do it's job? Remember, fevers over 105 degrees are rare. Have you ever had one that high? We are always scared and focused on the worst-case scenario, but these don't occur very often.

We have been trained to believe that our bodies are weak and that we should not trust our own innate intelligence. And so we pop pills. Tylenol, Advil, Pepto, Tums, Zyrtec, the list goes on and on. But do these pills make you healthy? Or do they cover up symptoms and make you "feel good" so that you can continue doing the things that caused the problem in the first place?

Your body is amazing! It has the potential to heal itself and it is constantly working to keep everything running inside you. Taking drugs to cover up or stop these processes is a bad idea. Of course there is the emergency situations where drugs and surgery are necessary, but again, these are rare.

When you have a headache, it is not because your body is deficient in Tylenol. Think about that. You might be dehydrated, lacking sleep, or just stressed out. Instead of popping a pill and banging away at whatever you were doing, why not take some time out and drink, rest, and relax. Take care of yourself. Excessive pill popping is a side effect of our go-go-go lifestyles. It isn't healthy.

16,000 people die every year from taking so-called "safe" drugs like Tylenol. You can look this information up on the CDC's website. Yet we start our kids on these pills from the moment of birth. It is no wonder we are seeing a rise in a myriad of health issues. Remember, there is always a trade-off in decisions you make that affect your health. A Tylenol today could mean kidney dysfunction tomorrow.

PUTTING IT ALL TOGETHER

Hopefully these pages have encouraged you to take steps towards living a healthier, more natural life. Hopefully you will look at the next health choice you encounter through the "lens of intended design" and more importantly trust yourself when you make the choice. As you know, chronic conditions like cancer, diabetes, and cardiovascular disease are on the rise. The generation of kids growing up right now is the first generation that, on average, will live a shorter life span than their parents. I see this statistic as a huge issue in our society, yet I remain optimistic because I am living proof that living a healthy lifestyle is attainable.

Living in optimal health is not as difficult as it seems. Remember to keep things simple and consider what our bodies were designed for. My personal journey has been successful because I used this lens to make logical choices about my health. I also attribute my success to taking things one step at a time. My new outlook on life and new habits took over a decade to develop. Give yourself permission to tackle one issue at a time, and give yourself permission to fail. If you miss a day at the gym or overindulge at a buffet, don't beat yourself up. Dust yourself off and get back with the program!

Don't be afraid to challenge or question "conventional wisdom". If that mode of thinking were working we would not be in this mess in the first place. Don't blindly swallow pills without asking if there is another way to achieve the end goal. You are your own best doctor and you are in charge of your health choices. Don't be afraid to get a second, third, or fourth opinion. Take as long as you need to find a doctor that understands you and is willing to work with you.

Your health is your most valuable asset and you need to invest in it every day. Without your health all of the material things you have accumulated mean nothing. It is time for a shift in your life; it is time to make health a priority.

Taking personal responsibility for your health is not the easy way. But when is the easy way the correct choice? I have never been able to come up with an example that shows the easy way is the right way. It is going to take some effort on your part, but never underestimate the power of your body.

Change seems difficult at first, but once a behavior becomes a habit you don't have to think about it anymore. So tackle things one at a time, when a behavior becomes a habit move on to the next goal. You will start to gain momentum and before you know it you will be a "health nut" too!

As I tell my children and as I tell myself, you are made of stardust and there are so many reasons for you to shine. Think about that for a second. Consider the amazing energy potential that is inside of you. The potential for health, the potential for love, the potential for achievement in your life. The only limitations are the ones you impose on yourself. Don't let conventional wisdom box you in.

www.ingramcontent.com/pod-product-compliance
Lightning Source LLC
Chambersburg PA
CBHW060636290526
45793CB00001B/266